THE SPANISH FLU PANDEMIC OF 1918

A True Story of the 1918 Influenza that devastated the World and What we can learn from it to Prepare for the Future

ANTHONY MORGAN

Copyright

Table of Contents

INTRODUCTION

Alfred Crosby said in his book "America's Forgotten Pandemic", that the important and almost unthinkable fact concerning the Spanish flu is that it killed millions of people in a year or less. There isn't any record in history - no infection, no war, no famine - that has ever killed so many in as short a period. And yet it has never inspired awe, not in 1918 and not since.

Epidemic diseases have typically altered the course of history, the death of a worldwide leader, an outbreak before a battle, however few diseases have accomplished it through sheer brute force.

The deadliest epidemic in history was neither smallpox nor the Black Death, it absolutely was the 1918 Spanish Flu.

In just one year, an estimated number of five hundred million people contracted the Spanish Flu worldwide, that was about a third of the world's population at that time. It killed between 50 to 100 million people, including some 675,000 Americans. In fact, the flu killed more Americans in a single year than in World War I, World War II, Korea, and Vietnam combined.

The 1918 flu was observed in Europe, the United States and parts of Asia before swiftly spreading around the world. At the time, medicine hasn't advanced yet- no effective drugs or vaccines were available to treat this killer flu strain.

States ordered their citizens to wear masks, social distancing was implemented - schools, theaters and businesses were closed.

This book will cover how the flu began and how it spread across the world, the bizarre symptoms that made it so deadly, measures and mistakes taken by some states in America and how the flu

pushed society to the very brink of collapse.

CHAPTER ONE

Spanish Flu Origin

No one can be absolutely sure where the pandemic originated but there are several theories; in northern France, there was an outbreak of a flu-like disease at a British military base in 1917. The base was located in a swampy area with lots of water farm and pigs. New flu epidemics often arise when people have close contact with sick birds or pigs.

There was a separate outbreak of respiratory disease among soldiers from Southeast Asia who fought in World War one (WWI) from 1916 to 1918. Most flus start in Southeast Asia and some historians argue the soldier may have brought a new virus to Europe.

Historian John Berry, makes the case in his fascinating book the great influenza that the flu may have originated on a farm in rural Kansas by jumping from infected pigs to humans.

Indeed, the first officially recognized cases of the Spanish flu emerged at a military base in Kansas, local physician Dr. Loring Miner saw dozens of his patients stricken by an unusually virulent form of flu in January to mid-March of 1918. The US had just entered World War one and training and industry had ramped up at a rapid pace as the war machine fired up. But in rural Haskel County Kansas, a war of another type was quietly beginning.

Haskell County was in the grip of a deadly outbreak of what seemed to be a mysterious new disease. People in the community, farmers mostly may have caught the new disease when a pathogen from sick pigs jumped species and began infecting humans. The new virus, the swine flu was shockingly contagious and extremely deadly. Dr. Miner was terrified by the death toll the new virus, that he contacted the US Public Health Service for advice, his concern was noted but nothing else was done. By the middle of March, the flu had faded away as quickly and as mysteriously as it had appeared. It might have ended, except for one unalterable fact – we were at war.

In early 1918 every military base was teeming with young men training for war, the military hurried to build new barracks, hospitals, training areas and facilities to support the influx of hundreds of thousands of men. Some of these men were volunteers and some had been drafted. The strange new disease was just dying down in Haskell County where few young men left there headed to camp Funston Kansas for training.

Camp Funston located at modern-day Fort Riley had a higher population than usual (about 56,000 young men) due to wartime training, there hadn't been time to build enough barracks for all of them. Because of the cold winter that year, soldiers were crowded together indoors with insufficient clothes and blankets, jammed closely around the few working stoves. Thereby violating the health and safety rules that dictated how much space each soldier should have inside the barracks.

Inside the barracks, men huddled around stoves trying to keep warm. The men from Haskell County must have crowded in close to even as they began to cough sneeze. That's all it took. In the overcrowded barracks the flu spread rapidly. It only took six days for the outbreak to begin. The men from Haskell County arrived on February 28th, less than one-week later men began to report to the infirmary with flu-like symptoms.

Within days, several thousand were stricken, killing between 38 and 50 – not enough to quarantine the camp in wartime. It was a high death rate for the flu but it was nothing compared to what was coming next. The virus was about to mutate and become much worse.

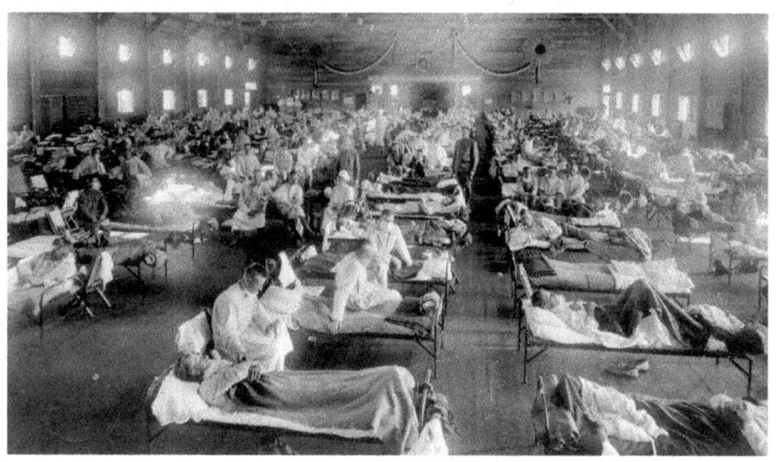
An emergency hospital during the influenza epidemic in Camp Funston, Kansas, via Wiki Commons

Flu viruses are constantly mutating and sometimes there will be a really big shift or a virus that usually affects the animals, mutate so it can infect people too. When that happens, it can be very deadly. The flu comes in waves that's why we have a flu season. Although it may seem like a bad flu is done, the flu can hide for a while or go infect people in a different part of the world and then return even worse.

In the case of the 1918 flu, three waves of flu devastated the world. The first wave wasn't too bad, that several doctors refused to believe it was even influenza. But the second and third waves were extremely dangerous. The outbreak at Camp Funston came just at the end of the flu season in the United States. So, the first wave infected a lot of people but then faded away. The military wasn't worried, they were grappling with the far more deadly outbreak of measles at the time. The flu virus seemed to fade away, but really it just went abroad to take on a world at war.

CHAPTER TWO

The Spread across Europe and beyond

Nearly all the ships carrying American troops to war arrived at the port in Brest France. In April of 1918, just as the flu outbreak was dying down at Camp Funston, an epidemic began in Brest and slowly began spreading throughout northern France. Despite the illness spreading in the city, more and more troops poured in. Healthy men would land, become infected and then ship out to new duty stations and to the frontline carrying the disease through every small town and hamlet through which the armies travelled.

The flu tour across France and followed the frontlines into Belgium and the Netherlands. It jumped across the lines of war and began infecting the German army, actually affecting the outcomes of battle since so many troops who were too sick to fight. It jumped from the German army to the German people, by May it reached Italy where it crossed the Mediterranean and surged into North Africa. it also arrived in England by May, riding back on boats with troops heading home. Infection and death rates began to skyrocket in Spain and Portugal.

The flu continued spreading beyond Western Europe, by July it had jumped to Scandinavian and Greece. The same month the flu crept its way into a tense Russia where the Tsar and his family had just been executed and the Bolsheviks were battling with other factions to see who would control the future of Russia.

A boat filled with six sailors arrived in Mumbai India at the end of May. First a few dock workers reported sick, then workers at the next docks became ill and then men at the nearby warehouses got sick and so on. Ships left those same infested docks and spread to other ports in

Asia, sick people boarded trains in Mumbai and spread the disease like wildfire along the railroad lines up into the subcontinent and continental Asia.

The flu showed up in China around the same time, spreading inland from a dock in Shanghai. By June, it had arrived in Singapore a world trade hub. The flu infected the dock workers and spread to the local population, from the bustling docks, sailors carried the flu south to Indonesia and north into Malaysia and Thailand where it continued to spread.

By July, it reached sub-Saharan Africa with infected sailors who arrived at the ports. It entered West Africa from ships arriving in Freetown Sierra Leone, it infected eastern Africa via the port in Mombasa Kenya. Ships arriving into Cape Town set the virus loose South Africa. From these ports, influenza ripped its way across the continent devastating the population

By July, it had also reached Peru and begun spreading across South America, by August it had returned to North America and it had reached New Zealand and Japan by October. A lethal outbreak was surging across Colombia, Argentina, Uruguay and Chile by November. Despite quarantines on ships entering port, dock restrictions and a concerted effort at containment, it finally spread into Australia by 1919.

In less than a year the deadly flu had surged around the world. The flu was able to spread so efficiently for many reasons including; the movement of vast companies of troops around the world and the conditions those troops were living in.

World War 1 was desperately brutal and trench warfare made for horrific living conditions and for the perfect breeding ground for disease. Men lived out in the open with no protection from the freezing winter, the pounding rain or the sweltering

Sun. Troops at the frontlines lived in filthy trenches for months at a time, where they had to eat sleep and answer all the calls of nature within close contact with each other.

When it rained, the trenches filled up with water that became foul as it had nowhere to drain. Soldier's feet rotted in their boots; a condition called trench foot. Dead bodies lay decomposing in no-man's land between the two armies. When it rained water would wash excrement, decomposing body parts and filth down into the trenches where the soldiers lived. Constant bombing turned up the dirt and turned the ground into a sloppy swamp, the mud became so bad that in some places it was like quicksand. Planks were laid down for the soldiers to walk on there.

By the end of the war, over 9 million combatants and 7 million civilians would die in the war. Thus, it's not surprising that when a violent new virus arrived, it became an even more deadly foe than the enemy soldiers.

Why Was It Called the Spanish Flu?

The flu gained its name, the Spanish flu, from the early infection and high mortality rate in Spain, where a reported eight million died in May. Spain was neutral in World War one and as a result it was one of the only countries that was reporting the news without strict government censorship. Most countries didn't want to reveal to their enemies that they were battling an epidemic and didn't want to affect their people's morale. So, the government pressured the media to hide and downplay the severity of the virus.

However, in neutral Spain the press was free to report the news accurately, newspaper headlines in Spain screamed of an epidemic that was killing millions. While other countries only whispered of the flu. The world believed the flu was worse in Spain when in actuality, Spain was the only Country talking about it at first.

CHAPTER THREE

Spanish Flu Symptoms

"We have had a number of cases where people were perfectly healthy and died within twelve hours."

- Charles Edward Winslow epidemiologist and professor at Yale University

At some point in the summer of 1918, the flu mutated to become more deadly. It gave some people the normal symptoms of fever, chills, nausea, aches and diarrhea. Many got sick then recovered like a normal flu. Some were sick longer or died after catching a secondary infection such as pneumonia.

However, many people became violently ill strange symptoms. In fact, in the July 1918 edition of the medical journal, the lancet doctors argued that this strange epidemic couldn't be the flu, because the symptoms didn't fit, Italian doctors argued the same.

In some people, Spanish flu cause fevers that were so high people hallucinated. Some cried of agonizing muscle pain so bad that doctors thought they had dengue also called break-bone fever. It made some people temporarily or even permanently blind, deaf or paralyzed. Some lost the ability to smell, some had strong vertigo and would fall over if they tried to walk.

Extreme ear infections developed very quickly, going from the first pain to the eardrums rupturing within only a few hours. Some had terrible headaches and double vision, severe mucus excretions and inflammation made it hard for victims to breathe. Some people coughed so hard they tore their abdominal muscles, Doctors doing autopsies saw lungs so damaged that they resembled those of people who died from poisonous gas and the war.

Some people developed a symptom most physicians had never seen before, tiny puffs of air would leak out from tears and lungs and get trapped beneath the skin, puffing up in little pockets all over their bodies. When they moved, the pockets would crackle like a bowl of rice crispies according to one nurse.

Some people developed hemorrhagic fever which like Ebola causes its victims to bleed. An army report described the flu as a rapidly escalating infection and lungs choked with blood fatal in from 24 to 48 hours. Some patients bled from their nose, their ears and their eyes.

Some victims with the 1918 flu, became so oxygen starved they began to turn blue or even looked black a condition called cyanosis. People reportedly turned so dark that it was difficult to distinguish white people from people of color. For this reason, the flu picked up the nickname the blue death and many wondered if the black death had returned.

When victims began turning blue, doctors knew they wouldn't survive more than a few hours. The flu was also terrifying because it could kill so quickly. Many victims died within a day or two or even hours of showing their first symptoms.

According to a story recounted in the book the great influenza, a man in Cape Town South Africa boarded a streetcar, just as a conductor died during the three-mile ride to his house six more people on the streetcar died. When the driver died, he got off the streetcar and walked home.

CHAPTER FOUR

The Second Wave

In late summer of 1918, the flu virus returned to America. But this time it was far more deadly. In August, a ship full of sick people arrived in a New York City from Europe. Four men had already died at sea and 200 more people on the ship were sick, many were taken to hospitals but they weren't quarantined. In the following week several more ships full of sick people arrived. The same was happening in other deep-water ports like; Boston, Philadelphia, New Orleans.

At the same time as the virus was arriving and spreading in ports, ships left those same ports headed for Canada, Central America, the Caribbean and South America carrying infected people. In early September, there was an outbreak at Navy Pier in Boston. The pier was quarantined but officers still moved between bases, an officer was probably responsible for carrying the flu to nearby camp Devens. At first just a few men reported sick and then within only a few days an epidemic broke out, by mid-September thousands of men were sick, in many cases violently so. Of those who were sick, seventy-five percent were so ill they had to be hospitalized.

The sheer number of patients overwhelmed the medical staff of the military hospital, the hospital had been designed to treat a maximum of 1200 troops at one time. Yet more than 6,000 patients were crammed in. Cots were stuffed into every available space in hallways and offices even on outdoor porches. The doctors and nurses felt ill, there were simply not enough healthy people to care for the thousands of sick people. So many died that they couldn't all fit in the hospital morgue, the dead were stacked up one on top of another like firewood in the hallway outside the morgue. Every day they were carted away and every day the hall filled up again.

The Army Medical Officers issued an order that no man should be sent to or shipped out of camp Devens, however, that's not what happened. A group of officers left camp Devens headed to Camp Grant in Illinois. Despite the rules against it, the chief officer there had authorized overcrowding due to a shortage in barracks. Once again giving the ideal environment for the disease to spread. Shortly after arriving, the officers from camp Devens became sick, the men were quarantined but it was already too late. Within two days of the first cases, the flu was widespread throughout the camp. Within four days of the first case, men started dying, within five days doctors and nurses became sick and started dying.

On the sixth day, there were 4,000 men admitted to the hospital and they converted ten barracks into temporary hospitals. By seven days, they were running out of Medicine, disinfectant and other medical supplies. By the ninth day, they converted nine more barracks to service hospitals bringing the number up to twenty. They didn't have enough beds sheets or ambulances to carry all the infirm, when they ran out of beds the soldiers were ordered to stuff straw into sacks to use as mattresses for the sick. Yet they still didn't have enough.

They tried to make enough face cloth to cover people's mouths to fight the spread of germs but they ran out of cloth. The Red Cross set up a station to notify relatives that their loved ones were dying or dead. Now relatives poured into the midst of a deadly epidemic, healthy relatives were escorted by coughing service members to identify dead bodies in the morgue. They crowded into the overfilled hospitals to visit a loved ones, desperate parents and wives tried to bribe nurses and orderlies to give special care to their soldier.

It became such a problem the head officer issued a warning about accepting bribes, those relatives would leave the camp and carry the infection out into the civilian community, into local towns on to cross-country trains and ultimately back to their own hometowns.

Civilian health officials called for an emergency quarantine of Camp Grant but the virus was already out. Four days after the first reported case a trainload of troops had left Camp Grant to go cross country to Camp Hancock near Augusta Georgia. For the journey of almost 1,000 miles the men were packed tightly into train cars with poor ventilation in the tight quarters. Men coughed, became feverish and began bleeding from their eyes and ears. They infected each other swiftly and the virus swept along the train, the train stopped repeatedly along the journey to refuel and the men who could still walk got off the train to get a break from the hacking coughs at the sick and delirious men.

There they interacted with railroad workers and curious locals who had come to see the troops, they infected town after town for almost 1,000 miles. When they finally arrived in Georgia, 2,000 of the 3,000 men were so sick they needed to be hospitalized immediately, they started a new outbreak at Camp Hancock. Historians don't know how many of the men from the train died, but one report from Fort Leonard Wood claims 10%. Yet when hundreds began dying, the medical staff at the hospital stopped keeping careful records, they were just too overwhelmed by all the dead.

CHAPTER FIVE

Philadelphia story

"I had a little bird its name was Enza. I opened the window and in-flu-enza."

- Children's jump-roping song, 1918.

The very worst outbreak probably occurred in Philadelphia and it was made immeasurably worse by mismanagement by leaders who ignored warnings from public health doctors. Had public health measures been implemented, perhaps much of the death and suffering could have been avoided.

Philadelphia in 1918 was teeming with people, hundreds of thousands had swarmed the city because of the new job opportunities; working at steel plants, docks, railroad yards and industries that supplied the war. Without enough housing for the influx, poor people were crowded into squalid filthy slums that lacked indoor plumbing. Multiple families would cram into one apartment and share an outhouse in an alleyway with hundreds of people. Sometimes people shared not only apartments but bed, even sleeping in ships.

The boarding houses would rent out beds for six or eight hours at a time, when one worker woke up to go to work another worker would get into the newly vacated bed and sleep, same sheets and all. The streets were notoriously filthy with rat infestations and gutters filled with trash, animal and even human feces. With people living in overcrowded conditions, exhausted from hard labor and weak from poor nutrition, dirty water and bad air quality, it was a perfect breeding ground for an epidemic.

A ship full of six sailors arrived into the Philadelphia Navy Yard in mid-September, within a few days the Navy hospital was overrun and the Navy began sending sailors to civilian hospitals in the city. As sailors began dying, the flu spread to civilians. Two days after the first sailor arrived at the hospital, multiple doctors and nurses felt fine as they started their shifts, yet collapsed and became desperately ill within hours.

However, the health board for the city didn't want people to panic, they downplayed the severity of the disease. After the death of several sailors and civilians, the Health Board confidently declared the disease had reached its peak and already begun to decline, when it hadn't even gotten started.

At the same time, the federal government was desperate for money from war bonds to fund the war. People would buy bonds essentially loaning the government money for a promise of being paid back later with interest.

Every city had a quota of bonds they had to sell and Philadelphia was ready to hold the Liberty loan parade to sell war bonds. Public health doctors begged the city to cancel the parade, terrified that it would cause the outbreak to become an epidemic. The city government ignored them.

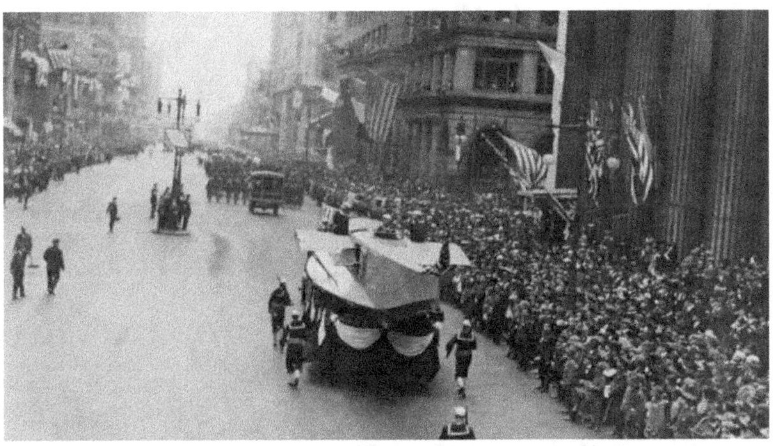

On September 28th, hundreds of thousands of people jammed into the downtown streets to watch the parade in that huddled crowd, all crushed together. It only took a few coughing, sneezing people to launch the epidemic. Within seventy-six hours just three days later, the city's 31 hospitals had run out of bed space. They were completely full, some hospitals tried to cram in more by laying patients on cots in the hallways, in offices and balconies. In some cases, the sick were laid on the floor next to a dying patient. Once the patient died, the body was taken away and the new patient will be lifted into the same bed still warm from the previous occupant.

The city opened several temporary emergency hospitals but it wasn't enough. Hospital started refusing to accept any more patients, people lined up outside begging to be let in. Some died standing in line, even for those who got in care was non-existent for most people. The hospitals ran out of Medicine, the doctors and nurses were overtasked and they were dropping from the flu. They were desperate for help people, with no medical training volunteered. Physicians and nurses came out of retirement, medical schools closed and third and fourth-year medical students were put in charge of an entire floor of a hospital.

One medical student reported that during the height of the outbreak, one-fourth of all the patients in the hospital died every day. Nurses were so overtasked they began adding toe tags to the living, so they could tag several at once. Once a patient turned blue, it was only a matter of hours to death. So, they felt confident in tagging them. Sometimes, there wasn't any time for an intervention, some people died within 24 hours of contracting them flu. A nurse at Mount Sinai Hospital started her shift in the morning and suddenly fell ill, she died 12 hours after first feeling sick.

The number of dead kept growing, five days after the city held the liberty loan parade, city leaders finally acted. The Health Department banned all public meetings, churches, schools and theaters were closed. They left the bars open.

The next day the courts closed and city services shut down. It took only a few days for the city's operations to completely grind to a halt. Within just 10 days, Philadelphia went from a few hundred cases of flu and a couple deaths per day to hundreds of thousands of people sick and hundreds dying every day, all because they ignored public health guidelines.

By the three weeks after the parade, the death toll stood at 4500. So many died that they could not be buried fast enough. Grave diggers were sick or refused to bury flu victims, the bodies started piling up inside morgues and funeral homes. Some Undertaker's raised their prices 500 percent to try and cash in, most ran out of coffins. One funeral home hired guards because people were trying to steal the coffins. People began wrapping their dead in blankets or sewing together flour sacks to use as shrouds. No one came to take the bodies and there was nowhere to bring them, so the dead stayed in the homes. people wrapped them in blankets.

Sometimes, people were so sick that the person in bed next to them would die and they couldn't gather the strength to take the body away. The city began to smell the stench of death hanging heavily in the air. Finally, families began digging their own graves to bury their dead.

Everyone was terrified, people avoided each other. There were cases of children whose parents got sick and the children starved because no one would go near them in case the child was sick. This was particularly a problem since those who were most likely to die were people aged between 20 to 40, many of them parents.

People couldn't get food because no trucks were delivering goods in the city, the streets fell silent, every business was closed, people hid inside their homes, the street cars stopped, the police cars stopped, the entire city ceased to function.

The Philadelphia city government was by now non-functional, wealthy Philadelphia families appealed to the federal government for help, but there was no help to send. Cities all across America were buckling beneath the weight of the epidemic and the federal government was busy managing the outbreak on military bases and among troops in Europe. With the city government failing to act, the women of elite Philadelphia families many of the same who had organized the Liberty loan parade, banded together to start outreach efforts. They gathered together civic leaders from across the city to start planning, they set up a special hotline to answer questions about the flu but had a hard time keeping it staffed because so many employees were sick.

They set up local neighborhood leaders, who would organize distribution of food and medical care. They also set up soup kitchens in the schools and food delivery to sick people as possible. Five hundred people volunteered their cars to be used as ambulances and to deliver food and drive doctors around a treat the sick. However, there was a desperate need for more volunteers and most people were too afraid to get involved. Leaders begged for more help but people turned away, the fabric of society began to break down.

City leaders who hadn't bothered to attend meetings of the outreach effort finally got involved. They seized the city's emergency fund to pay for supplies and pay health workers, they opened additional morgues and sent out policemen to try and clear the piled-up bodies. Like the ancient plagues, people carried their dead out to the streets. There the bodies were loaded onto open trucks or horse-drawn wagons, there were no coffins so they stack them one on top of the other.

By late October, the epidemic was finally beginning to loosen its death grip on the city. In its aftermath it left a death toll of 13,000, it also left thousands of orphaned children, a shortage of food and goods and a stalled city that had to slowly grind its most basic services back into motion.

CHAPTER SIX

How Other Cities Handled the Flu

"Phoenix are facing a crisis. Almost every home in the city has been stricken with the plague." - Arizona Republican November 8th 1918

In other cities and towns across America the news was the same, in New York City 33,000 people died before the statisticians stopped counting. Some small towns tried to keep the virus out by quarantine themselves, they shut down all businesses and canceled public gatherings. People were ordered to stay in their homes and not touch or visit others. Some towns made it illegal to shake hands, in other towns police were dispatched to nail signs on the doors of homes where people were sick. The sign said influenza in red letters.

Rumors spread in Phoenix Arizona that dogs spread the disease. Policemen killed dogs in the streets and people killed their own pets.

Colorado set up barricades on the roads and Men guarded them with shotguns, preventing anyone from coming in. Other towns couldn't stop the trains from rolling through in their local platforms, but they refused to let anyone step off the trains. Anyone who did was thrown in prison and quarantined. It didn't work, the virus still flipped in.

St. Louis Flattened the Infection Curve

Even before the first case of Spanish flu had been reported in the city, health commissioner Dr. Max Starkloff had local physicians on high alert and wrote an editorial in the St. Louis Post-Dispatch about the importance of avoiding crowds.

When a flu outbreak at a nearby military barracks first spread into the St. Louis civilian population, Starkloff wasted no time closing the schools, closing movie theaters and pool halls, and banned public gatherings of more than 20 people. These actions taken by Starkloff would later be known as social distancing.

There was pushback from business owners, but Starkloff and the mayor held their ground. When infections swelled as expected, thousands of sick residents were treated at home by a network of volunteer nurses.

All of the actions resulted in St. Louis experiencing one of the lowest influenza rates of cities compared to its size. Of the 31,500 who got sick in St. Louis only 1,703 died.

George Dehner, author of Global Flu and You: A History of Influenza, says that because of these precautions, St. Louis public health officials were able to "flatten the curve" and keep the flu epidemic from exploding overnight as it did in Philadelphia.

San Francisco Enforces Wearing Masks

A place that escaped the worst of the wrath was San Francisco and historians' credit that to aggressive response by the local government who listened to their public health officials. Public Health Director William Hassler, quarantined all naval stations before they had any reported cases. He ordered all public schools and gathering places closed, he divided the cities into separate districts with distinct support staff so as to segregate outbreaks. He also laid out plans and organized the flu response before the flu ever hit the city so they would be ready when it did.

The city's government medical and civic organizations banded together to educate citizens on prevention such as hand-washing, avoiding public places and wearing a face mask. While Philadelphia's government was still denying there was a problem, San Francisco authorities were distributing 100,000 face masks. Police enforced the facemask rule at gunpoint and actually shot people who refused to wear masks in the streets.

REFUSES TO DON INFLUENZA MASK; SHOT BY OFFICER

SAN FRANCISCO, Oct. 28.—While scores of passersby scurried for cover, H. D. Miller, a deputy health officer, shot and severely wounded James Wisser, a horseshoer, in front of a downtown drug store early today, following Wisser's refusal to don an influenza mask.

Accoerding to the police, Miller shot in the air when Wisser first refused his request. Wisser closed in on him and in the succeeding affray was shot in the arm and the leg.

Wisser was taken to the central emergency hospital, where he was placed under arrest for failure to comply with Miller's order.

As the second wave diminished throughout the country, San Francisco rejoiced for having missed the flu. The flu mutated once more and raged to the world for a third time, but infecting and killing fewer people. This time it would be less severe.

This time it did hit San Francisco because they thought the flu was already over. The third wave hit the South West and Midwest hard, before the rest of America the worst of the flu had passed.

Armistice Day and End of the Flu

Even as America woke from the nightmare the epidemic had left its imprint, right at the height of harvest time, farmers had been too sick to farm and workers didn't show up to gather the food in. Food that was harvested rotted in warehouses because there was no one to transport it. There was a lag while the country tried to catch up on shipping food and goods. Store shelves and markets stayed empty for some time because goods hadn't been delivered. As winter rolled in, there was a shortage of coal and other goods.

However, the weary country still rejoiced for an armistice was signed on November 11th 1918, the war was finally over.

By the summer of 1919, the flu pandemic came to an end, as those who were infected either died or developed immunity.

 In the US, the flu killed about 675000, the flu killed an estimated 3% of the entire world population. In Latin America, the flu killed 10 out of every 1,000 people.

In Africa about 15 out of every 1000 died and in parts of Asia the death rate was as high as 35 per thousand. In Tahiti it killed ten percent of the population and in Western Samoa twenty percent of the population died. In India alone, the flu killed about twenty million people.

CONCLUSION

Could there be another Pandemic?

You may be asking yourself, could a deadly flu like that happen again? it's important to understand that the Spanish flu was devastating for a number of reasons unique to that time.

However, the essential formula for epidemic still exists, viruses sometimes jump species. For instance, from pigs to human this could happen at any time anywhere in the world and of course flu viruses are constantly mutating.

Usually mutations are minor but occasionally a big mutation can happen. This has happened a few times in recent history, for instance the Russian flu of 1889 killed about 1 million people.

The Asian flu of 1957 killed about 2 million and the Hong Kong flu of 1968 also killed about 2 million. Then in 2018 exactly 100 years after the outbreak of Spanish flu, the mutation brought a particularly deadly flu to the US and Australia. As of 2018 there is one strain of avian flu, NH5 type that has managed to infect humans, but so far cannot jump between people.

However, that particular strain of flu is frightening in its potential according to Donald Burke MD, former director of the John Hopkins Center for immunization research. Of the people who have been affected, it has been deadly in over 75 percent of cases. If that type of flu adapted human to human infection it could be catastrophic.

The novel coronavirus pandemic of 2020 is spreading around the world as countries race to find a cure for COVID-19 and citizens shelter in place in an attempt to avoid spreading the disease, which is particularly deadly because many carriers are asymptomatic for days before realizing they are infected.

So, could it happen again? yes it could. Virtually every expert on influenza believes another pandemic is nearly inevitable, that it will kill millions of people, and that it could kill tens of millions — and a virus like 1918, or H5N1, might kill a hundred million or more — and that it could cause economic and social disruption on a massive scale.

As Burke said "when it comes to the probability of a pandemic flu, I think everyone would say, 'it's not if, it's when.'

REFERENCES

1. Remembering the 'Mother of All Pandemics,' 100 Years Later by Linda Poon - www.citylab.com/life/2018/09/spanish-flu-outbreak-1918-new-york-city-public-health-germ-city-museum/569947/

2. The Threat of Pandemic Influenza: Are We Ready?
https://www.nap.edu/read/11150/chapter/3

3. The Great Influenza: The Story of the Deadliest Pandemic in History by John M. Barry

4. Pale Rider: The Spanish Flu of 1918 and How It Changed the World by Laura Spinney

5. Spanish Flu - History.com Editors
https://www.history.com/topics/world-war-i/1918-flu-pandemic

9 7 9 8 6 3 7 5 8 6 2 5 7